LUNG TRANSPLANT POST DIET

A Comprehensive Guide To Nutritional Support, Optimizing Recovery, And Resillence In Respiration

DR LUCAS KAYCE

DISCLAIMER

This book about illness and nutrition is not meant to replace expert medical advice, diagnosis, or treatment; rather, it is meant purely for informational reasons. This book's content is founded on broad concepts and recommendations for managing diseases and nutrition.

Before adopting any major dietary or lifestyle changes, readers are recommended to speak with a qualified healthcare provider, such as a licensed physician or registered dietitian, especially if they have pre-existing medical concerns. Everybody has different health demands, so what works for one person might not work for another.

The use of the information provided in this book may have unfavorable repercussions or consequences, for which the author and publisher disclaim all liability. No disease is meant to be identified, treated, cured, or prevented by the information provided.

The book may include contain references to medical literature or research findings; however readers are urged to independently confirm this material and contact reliable sources.

It is important to remember that the fields of nutrition and medicine are always changing, and that new findings could have an impact on the advice offered in this book. As a result, readers are urged to keep up with the most recent advancements in healthcare and, when in doubt, seek professional counsel.

By reading this book, readers agree that they are in charge of their own health decisions and release the author and publisher from any liability arising from the use of the material in the book, whether direct or indirect.

TABLE OF CONTENTS

ABOUT THE BOOK

For those receiving a lung transplant, the book "Lung Transplant Post-Diet" is an excellent resource that provides thorough guidance on the critical post-transplant phase of treatment, with a focus on dietary considerations. A hearty welcome and acknowledgments are given in the opening section, which also sets the stage for a thorough examination of the topic.

The book set the stage by explaining the nuances of lung transplantation, such as its importance, signs, and the various kinds of transplant operations. It becomes critical for readers to comprehend the transplanting process to fully appreciate the nutritional recommendations that follow in the book.

The book explores the significance of a post-transplant diet, is a major emphasis point. This section outlines dietary restrictions and considerations that are essential for the best possible outcomes following a transplant, while also emphasizing the importance of nutrition in the healing process. It goes one step further, including advice on creating a nutritious diet after transplant, discussing the subtleties of balancing macronutrients, adding vitamins and micronutrients, and suggesting hydration intake.

The book covers practical elements in great detail, including meal planning advice and a repertory of recipes catered to post-transplant nutritional requirements. The book also offers advice on how to handle unusual dietary demands, including how to address food allergies and customize diets to meet specific needs.

There are specific sections on lifestyle and exercise, highlighting the value of physical activity following a lung transplant. This holistic approach goes beyond nutrition. Additionally it discusses the vital topic of emotional health, providing post-transplant patients with coping mechanisms for stress and anxiety as well as creating strong support networks.

The book wraps off with a focus on monitoring and follow-up, highlighting the importance of ongoing lab work, regular check-ups, and good contact with healthcare practitioners for long-term well-being. Essentially, "Lung Transplant Post-Diet" is an invaluable tool that combines medical knowledge with actionable advice to support people as they navigate the complex process of recovering from a lung transplant.

AN OVERVIEW OF TRANSPLANTING LUNGS

Over the years, lung transplantation has developed into a wonderful medical intervention for the treatment of severe respiratory disorders and ailments. A healthy lung from a deceased donor is used to replace a damaged or failing lung during this difficult surgical surgery. The goal is to restore adequate pulmonary function to prolong survival and improve the recipient's quality of life. Since its inception in the middle of the 20th century, lung transplantation has emerged as a promising treatment option for patients with end-stage lung conditions, including cystic fibrosis, idiopathic pulmonary fibrosis, and chronic obstructive pulmonary disease (COPD).

Sophisticated medical technologies and complex surgical techniques are used during the surgery to guarantee a successful lung transplant. Immunosuppressive drugs, postoperative care, and careful donor-recipient matching are essential steps in the process. To maximize results for the recipient, pulmonologists, surgeons, immunologists, and other healthcare specialists collaborate throughout the pre-transplant evaluation, transplant surgery, and recuperation period.

THE POST-TRANSPLANT DIET IS IMPORTANT

Moving on to the post-transplant phase, it is important to emphasize the need for a carefully planned and supervised post-transplant diet. The function that the post-transplant diet plays in promoting the transplant recipient's general health and impacting the transplant's outcome makes it significant. During the recovery phase, the body's nutritional requirements alter significantly, and a well-planned diet becomes essential for immune system function, the healing process, and avoiding problems.

Considerations for a post-transplant diet go beyond calorie consumption. Foods high in nutrients and vitamin and mineral supplements are essential for supporting the recipient's immune system, which is frequently weakened by immunosuppressive drugs used to stop organ rejection. Nutritionists and other healthcare professionals must closely monitor patients to ensure that the delicate work of balancing providing dietary demands with preventing potential medication interactions is accomplished.

In addition, the management of possible consequences including weight gain, diabetes, and hypertension—which can result from side effects of both the transplant procedure and the accompanying medications—is also impacted by the significance of the post-transplant diet. In addition to helping to avoid these issues, a well-managed diet also improves the recipient's general health and makes the shift to a more active and healthy lifestyle easier.

Lung transplantation provides a ray of hope for those suffering from serious lung conditions, providing a possibility for a better quality of life and a longer survival time. However, the effectiveness of this medical intervention depends on comprehensive care given during the post-transplant period as well as surgical skills and pre-transplant examinations. Ensuring the overall health and well-being of the transplant recipient requires acknowledging the significance of a customized post-transplant diet as a crucial component of the healing process.

CHAPTER ONE

COMPREHENDING LUNG TRANSPLANTATION

LUNG TRANSPLANTATION: WHAT IS IT?

The goal of a lung transplant is to use a donor lung that is healthy to replace a damaged or failing lung. When alternative forms of treatment for serious lung problems have failed, consideration is usually given to this intricate and potentially life-saving surgical procedure. Enhancing the patient's quality of life and chances of survival is the ultimate aim of lung transplantation.

GUIDELINES FOR LUNG TRANSPLANTATION

Lung transplants can be indicated for a variety of conditions, most commonly end-stage lung disorders. Idiopathic pulmonary fibrosis, cystic fibrosis, chronic obstructive pulmonary disease (COPD), and pulmonary hypertension are common disorders that may require a lung transplant. Lung function frequently declines significantly in patients with these disorders, resulting in severe symptoms and a shorter life expectancy. When medical treatment and other measures are no longer able to control the underlying lung disease's progression, lung transplantation becomes a feasible alternative.

LUNG TRANSPLANT TYPES

Lung transplants come in a variety of forms, each suited to the patient's unique requirements. Single lung transplantation and double lung transplantation are the two main varieties.

In a single lung transplant, a healthy donor lung is used to replace the diseased lung, whereas in a double lung transplant, both lungs are replaced. The patient's general health status, the kind and severity of the lung illness and the availability of donor organs all play a role in the decision between these treatments. Another variation is heart-lung transplantation, which involves the simultaneous transplanting of the heart and lungs and is usually recommended for certain heart and lung diseases.

THE PROCEDURE FOR TRANSPLANTATION

The transplant procedure is a rigorously regulated, multi-professional endeavor that follows strict guidelines. A thorough assessment of the patient's medical background, present state of health, and degree of lung illness is the first step in the procedure. When a patient is declared transplantable, they are added to a waiting list for a suitable donor organ. Blood type, size, and medical urgency are among the considerations that go into determining organ allocation.

The transplant procedure is carried out once a qualified donor is found. The surgical team replaces the damaged lung or lung(s) with the donor lung or lung(s). The actual procedure is complex, requiring close attention to detail to guarantee the transplanted organ(s) attach and operate properly. Patients are kept under constant observation and undergo intensive care following the treatment to control any complications and guarantee a speedy recovery.

Recipients of transplants need to take immunosuppressive drugs for the rest of their lives to prevent organ rejection. By inhibiting the immune system's reaction, these drugs lessen the possibility that the body may attack and harm the transplanted lung or lung(s). To evaluate the functioning of the transplanted lung or lung(s) and swiftly address any possible problems, routine follow-up appointments and monitoring are crucial. lung transplantation is an essential treatment for people with severe, terminal lung illnesses. The ultimate goal of increasing the patient's quality of life and prolonging their survival is carefully considered when deciding whether to receive a lung transplant. Potential hazards and advantages are also carefully considered. Collaboration between medical staff, patients, and their support systems is essential for the successful outcome of lung transplants, and it emphasizes the significance of continued care and following post-transplant guidelines.

CHAPTER TWO

GUIDELINES FOR POST-TRANSPLANT NUTRITION

NUTRITION IS IMPORTANT AFTER LUNG TRANSPLANT

Sustaining proper nutrition becomes critical for the recipient's general health and speedy recovery following lung transplant surgery. It is impossible to overestimate the significance of diet following a lung transplant since it is essential for promoting the body's healing process, boosting immunity, and avoiding problems. Sufficient nourishment is crucial for tissue regeneration, maintaining organ function, and reducing the stress the body experiences during transplant surgery and the healing phase.

DIETARY LIMITATIONS AND THINGS TO THINK ABOUT

Following particular dietary requirements and limits is one of the most important things to consider for persons who have had a lung transplant. These rules are intended to reduce the possibility of issues and guarantee that the new organ performs at its best. Typical dietary restrictions include limiting salt intake to control blood pressure and avoiding specific foods that could interfere with immunosuppressive drugs. Due to the increased susceptibility of immunosuppressed individuals to opportunistic pathogens, patients are frequently recommended to avoid eating raw or undercooked food to reduce their risk of infection.

Post-transplant patients need to be aware of dietary restrictions as well as other factors that could affect how much nutrients they consume. Nutritional decisions can be influenced by drug interactions, possible pharmaceutical adverse effects, and metabolic changes. Healthcare practitioners must examine patients regularly to modify nutritional regimens according to individual demands and growing health issues. Dietitians and transplant teams must work together to provide a comprehensive approach to the patient's care.

NUTRITIONAL OBJECTIVES FOR PATIENTS AFTER TRANSPLANTATION

Post-transplant patients have a variety of nutritional needs that are targeted at meeting their needs for long-term recovery and well-being. Sustaining a sufficient intake of calories is essential to meet the body's heightened energy needs while it heals.

Patients may have muscle atrophy during the recovery phase, therefore maintaining muscle mass and repairing damaged tissue require enough protein intake. To maintain immunological function and general health, micronutrient requirements, such as those for vitamins and minerals, are also closely watched.

Another essential component of post-transplant nutrition is hydration. For drug absorption, organ function, and the avoidance of consequences such as renal problems, proper fluid balance is crucial. Healthcare professionals frequently advise patients on the proper amounts of fluid intake while taking into account their unique medical conditions and prescription needs.

Sustaining optimum nutrition throughout the post-transplant period has specific problems and considerations. It is impossible to overestimate the significance of following dietary recommendations, overcoming constraints, and pursuing certain nutritional objectives. To guarantee the greatest outcomes for patients who have had lung transplants, a comprehensive strategy involving cooperation between medical professionals, transplant teams, and nutritionists is necessary. A well-designed and monitored nutritional plan can help patients heal more quickly, experience fewer side effects, and have a happier life after transplantation.

CHAPTER THREE

CREATING A HEALTHFUL DIET FOLLOWING A TRANSPLANT

PROPER MACRONUTRIENT BALANCE

The careful balancing of macronutrients (carbs, proteins, and fats) is an essential part of a good post-transplant diet. The amounts of each macronutrient in the diet have a substantial impact on general health, and each one supports the body's functioning differently.

A balanced diet is crucial for transplant recipients to assist their body's healing, maintain ideal energy levels, and enhance their general well-being.

Since they are the main source of energy, carbohydrates have to make up a sizable amount of a post-transplant diet. Excellent sources of complex carbs that also provide necessary nutrients and dietary fiber are whole grains, fruits, and vegetables. For transplant recipients who want to maintain a healthy lifestyle, weight management is a critical factor that this fiber can help with. It is also helpful for digestive health.

Proteins are essential for the healing process following a transplant because they are involved in immunological response and tissue repair. Lean protein sources include beans, fish, chicken, and low-fat dairy products can be included to assist satisfy these dietary requirements. Consuming enough protein aids in the recovery process and prevents the loss of muscle, which is crucial for people recovering from surgery.

Fats are necessary for the creation of hormones and the absorption of nutrients, but they should only be eaten in moderation. Choosing heart-healthy fats from foods like olive oil, avocados, nuts, and seeds can enhance a well-balanced diet without jeopardizing cardiovascular health.

To meet their nutritional needs and maintain general health, recipients of transplants should concentrate on ensuring a balanced intake of all three macronutrients.

SUPPLEMENTS AND MICRONUTRIENTS

Transplant recipients need to be particularly aware of micronutrients, which are vitamins and minerals that are essential for several physiological processes, in addition to macronutrients. Sustaining the immune system, guarding against deficiencies, and fostering maximum health all depend on maintaining an adequate supply of vitamins and minerals.

Micronutrient-dense fruits and vegetables include minerals like potassium and magnesium along with vitamins A, C, and K. A wide range of vital nutrients can be included in the post-transplant diet with the support of a colorful and varied assortment of plant-based foods.

To support the body's demands during the healing process or to address any shortages, medical practitioners may occasionally suggest certain supplements. For transplant recipients, vitamin D, calcium, iron, and B vitamins are common supplements. Before adding supplements to their regimen, people should, however, speak with their healthcare provider because taking too much of some vitamins and minerals might have negative consequences.

FLUID CONSUMPTION SUGGESTIONS

For individuals recovering from transplants, staying properly hydrated is essential to supporting kidney function and general health. Consuming the recommended amount of fluids keeps the body from becoming dehydrated, supports healthy organ function, and facilitates the body's removal of waste.

The most common and organic option for hydration is water. Individual demands, activity levels, and weather conditions should all be taken into consideration when determining the appropriate amount of water to consume during the day for transplant recipients. Urine color can be used as a straightforward indicator of one's level of hydration; a light yellow or straw color indicates sufficient hydration.

Transplant recipients should be aware of the total amount of fluid in their diet, which includes soups, fruits, and vegetables, even if water is the recommended beverage. But it's important to keep the amount of sugary and caffeinated drinks you consume to a minimum because too much of either can cause dehydration and have a detrimental effect on your general health.

The amount of fluid that each person needs can vary depending on their age, weight, medications, and renal function. Thus, to promote their continued recovery and well-being, transplant recipients should collaborate closely with their healthcare team to identify tailored recommendations for fluid intake and make any adjustments.

CHAPTER FOUR

RECIPES AND MEAL PLANNING

MAKING WELL-COMPOSED MEALS

Developing well-balanced meals is essential to keeping a diet that is both healthful and comprehensive. A range of vitamins and minerals are often included in a balanced meal, along with macronutrients including proteins, lipids, and carbohydrates. This method guarantees that the body gets the nutrition it needs to function at its best. People should include a variety of foods from various food categories in their meals to attain balance.

To begin, incorporate a range of vibrant fruits and vegetables into your meals. These supply vital minerals, vitamins, and antioxidants. Whole grains are great sources of complex carbs that provide long-lasting energy. Examples of these are quinoa, brown rice, and whole wheat. Lean protein sources, such as fish, chicken, beans, and tofu, aid in the upkeep and repair of muscles. Nuts, avocados, and olive oil are good sources of healthy fats that support several body processes, including hormone balance.

When it comes to meal planning, having well-balanced plans is essential to ensuring that nutritional demands are met throughout the day or week. A well-organized meal plan considers lifestyle variables, nutritional needs, and personal food preferences. It frequently entails distributing nutrition throughout the day to sustain energy levels and avoid overindulging in any particular meal.

EXAMPLE MENUS

Meal plan examples can be useful tools for people who want to make dietary decisions more efficiently. These programs can be adjusted to meet different calorie requirements and dietary preferences, such as being gluten-free or vegetarian. A well-rounded dinner that incorporates a range of food groups, a nutrient-dense lunch consisting of lean proteins and vegetables, and a balanced breakfast consisting of whole grains, proteins, and fruits could be included in a normal day's meal plan. Strategic inclusion of snacks can help sustain energy levels in between meals.

Making thoughtful dietary decisions is essential for aiding the healing process and general health of those following a transplant. In these situations, meal planning must consider certain dietary requirements or advice from medical specialists. Nutrient-dense food consumption becomes crucial for tissue repair, since protein intake may be especially vital. Lean meats, whole grains, and a range of fruits and vegetables can all assist supply the vital elements required for a diet following transplantation.

RECIPES FOR A DIET AFTER TRANSPLANTATION

Recipes for a post-transplant diet should emphasize foods that are high in vitamins and minerals, low in sodium, and simple to digest. Quinoa and steamed veggies go well with lean proteins like chicken or fish that are baked or grilled. Vegetables and lean proteins together can make for nutrient-dense, easily modifiable soups and stews. Smoothies made with yogurt, fruits, and protein sources can be a delightful and practical choice.

Panning balanced meals requires carefully taking into account different dietary groups and nutrients. For example, meal plans serve as useful resources for incorporating a healthy diet into day-to-day activities. It's critical to modify recipes to suit the individual nutritional requirements of people following a transplant to promote healing and general well-being.

HANDLING FOOD ALLERGIES AND SPECIAL DIETARY NEEDS

Taking care of food allergies is a crucial part of managing specific dietary needs. Food allergies must be properly identified and managed because they can provide major health hazards. Comprehending the particular allergens that cause reactions in individuals is essential because it makes it possible to design individualized diet programs that either exclude or replace substances that cause issues. To protect the safety of those with allergies, common allergens like nuts, shellfish, dairy, and gluten must be carefully considered when meal planning and cross-contamination hazards should be kept to a minimum.

CUSTOMIZING THE DIET TO MEET SPECIFIC NEEDS

Managing unique dietary requirements requires individualization, and establishing diets that are tailored to a person's needs is essential to fostering optimum health. Creating customized meal plans involves taking into account several variables, including age, health issues, cultural preferences, and personal tastes. Dietary adjustments are necessary for people with medical disorders such as diabetes, hypertension, or celiac disease to regulate blood pressure, control blood sugar levels, or stay away from gluten-containing foods. Working together with dietitians and medical specialists is essential to creating diet plans that fit individual preferences and lifestyles in addition to meeting nutritional demands.

TAKING CARE OF COMMON DIETARY CHALLENGES

Taking care of specific dietary demands frequently entails taking care of common food issues that people could run into. One of these difficulties is continuing to eat a varied and well-balanced diet while following certain guidelines. For instance, to maintain appropriate bone health, people who are lactose intolerant may need to find alternate sources of calcium and vitamin D. It's also critical to overcome the psychological and social components of dietary constraints. People with unique dietary needs may face difficulties at social gatherings and festivities. It helps to foster a supportive environment and guarantees that dietary restrictions are adhered to when affected persons and those around them are informed about the dietary requirements.

CHAPTER FIVE

LIFESTYLE AND EXERCISE

THE BENEFITS OF EXERCISE FOLLOWING A LUNG TRANSPLANT

Exercise is essential to the recovery process and general well-being of people who have had this life-altering surgery. It also plays a major role in the post-lung transplant journey. Maintaining a healthy body weight, strengthening lung function, and promoting cardiovascular health are just a few of the benefits of regular physical activity. Patients frequently see improvements in their ability to breathe after receiving a lung transplant, and adding exercise to their daily routine helps to maximize these changes.

The beneficial effects of physical activity on cardiovascular health are among the main advantages following a lung transplant. The benefits of exercise for transplant recipients include improved blood circulation, a stronger heart, and assistance in controlling blood pressure.

Regular exercise also helps avoid complications like blood clots and cardiovascular disorders, which is especially advantageous for those who may have struggled with these issues before receiving a transplant.

INCLUDING EXERCISE IN EVERYDAY ACTIVITIES

A vital component of keeping up a healthy lifestyle after a lung transplant is incorporating exercise into everyday activities. To reap the long-term benefits, physical activity must become a regular part of one's lifestyle. Depending on personal preferences and fitness levels, this might encompass a range of activities from low-impact workouts like swimming and walking to more strenuous workouts.

Developing a long-term fitness regimen benefits mental health as well as physical health by assisting people in managing the psychological and emotional components of their recovery.

MANAGING EXERCISE AND SLEEP

Finding a healthy mix between rest and movement is essential for people recovering from lung transplants. As crucial as exercise is, it's also critical to understand when you need to rest and recover. Excessive effort might cause exhaustion and hinder the healing process. Finding the ideal balance requires paying attention to one's body, being aware of one's limitations, and modifying the volume and duration of physical activity as necessary.

This harmony guarantees that people can get the rewards of physical activity without sacrificing their general well-being and recuperation.

Moreover, there are more advantages to exercise than only improved physical health when incorporated into daily life after transplant. It offers a chance for social interaction, fostering a sense of belonging and support. Participating in sports, walks, or group workouts can help transplant recipients interact with people who may have gone through similar things. This can create a supporting network that improves their general well-being.

It is impossible to exaggerate the value of exercise following a lung transplant. It is a vital component of post-transplant treatment, supporting respiratory health, cardiovascular health, and general well-being. A deliberate and balanced strategy is needed to incorporate exercise into daily living, taking into account each person's level of fitness and need for relaxation. By preserving this balance, people can speed up their recuperation, get the psychological and physical rewards of exercise, and create a community of support that enriches their experience after receiving a transplant.

CHAPTER SIX

PSYCHOLOGICAL WELLNESS

HANDLING STRESS AND ANXIETY

Managing stress and anxiety is essential to preserving mental health. Although stress and worry are normal reactions to difficult circumstances, prolonged or excessive stress can be harmful to one's mental health. Acquiring efficient coping strategies is crucial for managing life's unavoidable challenges. Deep breathing exercises and other mindfulness techniques, which support calmness and lessen the body's reaction to stress, are common sources of relief for people. In addition, eating a balanced diet, getting enough sleep, and exercising frequently are all essential components of stress and anxiety management.

Seeking expert assistance through counseling or therapy can offer helpful coping mechanisms and techniques for handling these difficulties, promoting long-term emotional resilience.

SUPPORT NETWORKS FOR TRANSPLANT PATIENTS

During their recuperation, transplant recipients may confront particular emotional difficulties. Stress and anxiety levels can rise as a result of the transplant process's psychological and physical costs as well as the unpredictability of the results. Creating strong support networks is essential to assisting patients in overcoming these obstacles.

Friends and family are invaluable sources of understanding, encouragement, and emotional support. Support groups designed with transplant recipients in mind can provide a sense of belonging and common experiences. A key component of providing comprehensive treatment is the healthcare team, which includes mental health and transplant coordinators.

It is essential to treat the psychological as well as the physical components of healing to promote a comprehensive and fruitful post-transplant experience.

MENTAL HEALTH AND RECOVERY

Several facets of general well-being are associated with the confluence of mental health and recovery. Recovering from a physical ailment, an addiction, or a traumatic experience is closely associated with mental health. A thorough rehabilitation strategy must recognize and treat mental health concerns. Mental health issues might impede the healing process by taking the form of anxiety, sadness, or post-traumatic stress disorder. Rehab strategies must include mental health services to foster resilience and avoid recurrence. Psychotherapy and counseling are examples of therapeutic procedures that can give people the skills they need to deal with difficult emotions and create coping mechanisms. In addition, creating a community atmosphere that is accepting and encouraging helps to lower stigma and promote candid discussions about mental health, creating a climate in which people feel empowered to give their emotional health priority while they go through recovery.

CHAPTER SEVEN

MONITORING AND SUSTAINING

FREQUENT MEDICAL EXAMINATIONS

Preventive healthcare relies heavily on routine health examinations, which operate as proactive steps to identify and treat potential health problems before they worsen. These standard exams, which are usually carried out by medical specialists, comprise a thorough evaluation of a person's general state of health. Frequent examinations facilitate the early detection of risk factors, allowing for prompt interventions and individualized treatment regimens. Detailed vital sign examinations, reviews of medical histories, and discussions about lifestyle factors that may affect health are frequently included in these visits.

LAB EXAMINATIONS AND TRACKING PARAMETERS

Lab testing and parameter monitoring are essential components of the continuous evaluation of an individual's health. These examinations offer unbiased information on a range of physiological and biochemical indicators, shedding light on blood chemistry, organ function, and any anomalies. Healthcare professionals can make well-informed decisions about diagnosis and treatment by analyzing changes over time in factors like blood pressure, cholesterol, blood glucose, and others. For those with chronic diseases in particular, routine monitoring are crucial because it enables treatment plans to be modified in response to changing health dynamics.

INTERACTING WITH HEALTHCARE PROFESSIONALS

Having efficient communication with medical professionals is essential to continuing to deliver thorough and customized care. To ensure a full knowledge of health issues, treatment alternatives, and follow-up plans, patients and healthcare practitioners need to have open and transparent discussions. People are empowered to actively participate in their healthcare decisions when there is clear communication, which cultivates a collaborative partnership. Additionally, it makes it possible for medical professionals to customize therapies according to the needs and desires of the patient, promoting a patient-centered care philosophy.

It is the duty of both patients and healthcare practitioners to be informed about a patient's health state in the context of monitoring and follow-up. Frequent health examinations provide the chance to talk about changing one's lifestyle, taking prescription drugs as directed, and coming up with new plans to improve one's health. When read in conjunction with clinical assessments, lab test results offer objective facts that help create a comprehensive understanding of a person's health.

Furthermore, answering queries and addressing concerns are equally important components of good communication as information sharing. It should be easy for patients to voice their opinions, seek clarification, and offer comments regarding their experiences with healthcare management. Conversely, medical professionals should actively listen to patients, make difficult medical concepts clear, and promote patient participation in their treatment plans.

Routine physical examinations, laboratory examinations, and efficient correspondence with medical professionals are essential elements of observation and subsequent care in the medical field. These procedures aid in the continual evaluation of physiological data, the early identification of health problems, and the development of cooperative partnerships between patients and medical staff. People can actively participate in their healthcare by giving these factors priority, which will improve results and quality of life.